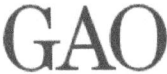

United States Government Accountability Office

Report to Congressional Requesters

I0448119

May 2013

HOMELAND SECURITY

An Overall Strategy Is Needed to Strengthen Disease Surveillance in Livestock and Poultry

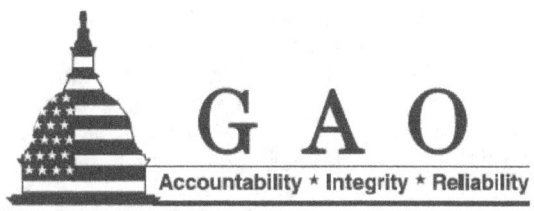

GAO
Accountability * Integrity * Reliability

GAO-13-424

Highlights of GAO-13-424, a report to congressional requesters

HOMELAND SECURITY

An Overall Strategy Is Needed to Strengthen Disease Surveillance in Livestock and Poultry

Why GAO Did This Study

International animal health authorities have stated that disease surveillance in livestock and poultry has as its main purpose the early detection of diseases and disease outbreaks. APHIS has worked closely with states and industry over the past decades to eradicate diseases by, for example, providing states with funding and guidance. But the disease landscape has changed, with rapid global movement of humans and animals, creating new threats. GAO was asked to review federal animal disease surveillance efforts. This report examines (1) USDA's new approach to disease surveillance in light of a changing disease landscape and challenges, if any, the agency faces with this approach and (2) the extent to which this approach is guided by a strategy with measurable goals and supports broader national biosurveillance efforts. GAO reviewed relevant presidential directives, laws, regulations, guidance, policies, documents, and strategic plans related to disease surveillance in animals; visited swine facilities; and interviewed federal, state, and industry veterinarians and other officials.

What GAO Recommends

GAO recommends that as APHIS develops goals and measures for its new approach, it integrate the agency's vision into an overall strategy guiding how this approach supports national homeland security efforts to enhance the detection of biological threats. In their comments, USDA concurred with GAO's recommendation, and the Department of Homeland Security described its commitment to disease surveillance efforts.

View GAO-13-424. For more information, contact Daniel Garcia-Diaz, (202) 512-3841 or garciadiazd@gao.gov.

What GAO Found

Under a new approach, the U.S. Department of Agriculture's (USDA) Animal and Plant Health Inspection Service (APHIS) has begun broadening its previous disease-by-disease approach to disease surveillance to one in which the agency monitors the overall health of livestock and poultry and uses additional sources and types of data to better detect and control new or reemerging diseases. APHIS's first effort under its new approach is to monitor the health of the nation's swine herds and identify new sources and types of data on diseases in swine, among other things. In planning documents, APHIS officials have proposed collecting data from farms where swine are raised, markets where they are sold, slaughter facilities, and veterinary diagnostic laboratories, among other sites. For example, APHIS has been monitoring for the presence of pseudorabies—a viral disease of swine that may cause respiratory illness and death—at slaughter facilities, but under the new approach, it has proposed monitoring these facilities for a range of other diseases as well. Key challenges to carrying out this new approach are how best to obtain data from producers, who are concerned that health information about their herds and flocks be kept confidential, and how to obtain health data in sufficient quantity from some animals like feral swine. Resource constraints also present a challenge, according to agency and state officials, given the recent decrease in APHIS's budget of about 14 percent for fiscal years 2008 through 2013.

APHIS has a vision for its new approach but has not integrated that vision into an overall strategy with associated goals and performance measures that are aligned with the nation's larger biosurveillance efforts. The Government Performance and Results Act, as amended, requires federal agencies to develop performance plans that include goals and performance measures. GAO has previously reported that these requirements can also serve as leading practices for planning at lower levels within agencies, such as individual divisions or programs. Developing goals and measures helps an organization balance competing priorities, particularly if resources are constrained, and helps an agency assess progress toward intended results. APHIS has developed a number of planning documents related to the agency's capabilities in disease surveillance in livestock and poultry, which acknowledge that the agency plays an important role in safeguarding public and environmental health. Goals APHIS has identified in these documents, however, focus primarily on processes or activities and do not specifically address outcomes the agency seeks to accomplish or have associated performance measures. Moreover, none of the planning documents indicate how they individually or collectively support national homeland security efforts called for in Homeland Security Presidential Directive 9, which assigns several federal agencies, including USDA, responsibility for establishing a comprehensive and coordinated surveillance system to support early detection of biological threats, including infectious diseases. Agency officials said they plan to develop goals and measures for the new approach. Without integrating its vision into an overall strategy with goals and measures aligned with broader national homeland security efforts to detect biological threats, APHIS may not be ideally positioned to support national efforts to address the next threat to animal and human health.

Contents

Tables

Figures

Abbreviations

APHIS	Animal and Plant Health Inspection Service
CDC	Centers for Disease Control and Prevention
HHS	Department of Health and Human Services
OIE	World Organisation for Animal Health
USDA	U.S. Department of Agriculture

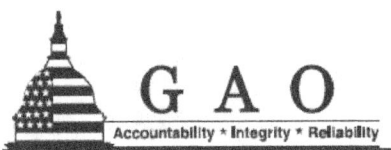
May 21, 2013

The Honorable Susan W. Brooks
Chairman
Subcommittee on Emergency Preparedness, Response, and
Communications
Committee on Homeland Security
House of Representatives

The Honorable Gus M. Bilirakis
House of Representatives

The agricultural sector is a critical component of the nation's
infrastructure. Threats to the sector may not only sicken animals used for
food but also seriously harm the economy and human health. A 2001
outbreak of foot-and-mouth disease in the United Kingdom, for example,
resulted in the slaughter of more than 4 million animals to contain the
disease, losses of over $5 billion to the food and agriculture sectors, and
comparable losses to the tourism industry.[1] In addition, physical
boundaries have narrowed between expanding human populations,
wildlife, and commercial agriculture, and technological advances have
facilitated the rapid movement of humans, animals, and food products
around the world. As these boundaries have narrowed and these
technological advances have taken place, the landscape for animal and
human disease and its associated surveillance—that is, the process of
collecting, analyzing, and exchanging information related to cases of
infectious diseases—has also changed. In fact, the National Academies
report that nearly two-thirds of infectious diseases affecting humans result
from pathogens transmitted between animals and people, causing

---

[1]We have reported that foot-and-mouth disease is a highly contagious viral disease of
cloven-hoofed animals, such as cattle, swine, and sheep. Infected animals develop a fever
and blisters on their tongues, lips, and between their hooves. Many animals recover from
a foot-and-mouth disease infection, but the disease leaves them debilitated and causes
losses in meat and milk production. Foot-and-mouth disease does not have human health
implications. It can be spread by animals, people, or materials that bring the virus into
physical contact with susceptible animals. The disease is also considered a potential
agent for agroterrorism. A foot-and-mouth disease outbreak has not occurred in the United
States since 1929, although the disease is considered widespread in parts of Africa, Asia,
Europe, and South America. See GAO, *Homeland Security: Actions Needed to Improve
Response to Potential Terrorist Attacks and Natural Disasters Affecting Food and
Agriculture*, GAO-11-652 (Washington, D.C.: Aug. 19, 2011).

diseases known as zoonoses. Under this changing disease landscape, not only can the emergence of a single, highly contagious animal disease bring sales of livestock and poultry to a standstill, but a pathogen that is transmissible to humans who lack immunity can also have wide impact on public health. The 2009 novel H1N1 influenza virus with origins in swine is one example of a recent mutation of an influenza virus that affected both human health and the pork industry, a vital part of U.S. agriculture. Not only did the virus cause a worldwide influenza epidemic, or pandemic,[2] but it also led to substantial losses in pork sales when consumers mistakenly believed they could become infected by eating pork.

To establish a national policy to defend against, among other threats, potentially catastrophic effects of disease outbreaks in animals, the President issued Homeland Security Presidential Directive 9 in 2004. This directive assigns to several federal agencies—including the U.S. Department of Agriculture (USDA) and the Department of Health and Human Services—responsibility for establishing a comprehensive and coordinated surveillance system to support early detection of infectious diseases, among other things. Also under presidential directive 9, the Department of Homeland Security shall coordinate with appropriate federal agencies to create a new biological threat awareness capacity to enhance detection and characterization of an attack.[3] USDA exercises its authority under the Animal Health Protection Act to detect, control, and eradicate diseases in livestock and poultry through its Animal and Plant Health Inspection Service (APHIS).[4] In addition, the Centers for Disease Control and Prevention (CDC), within the Department of Health and Human Services, has entered into a collaborative agreement to work with

---

[2]GAO, *Influenza Pandemic: Lessons from the H1N1 Pandemic Should Be Incorporated into Future Planning,* GAO-11-632 (Washington, D.C.: June 27, 2011).

[3]The Department of Homeland Security has defined *biosurveillance* as "the science and practice of managing human, animal, plant, food, and environmental health-related data and information for early warning of threats and hazards, early detection of events, and rapid characterization of the event so that effective actions can be taken to mitigate adverse health, social, and economic effects." See Department of Health and Human Services, Centers for Disease Control and Prevention, *National Biosurveillance Strategy for Human Health,* version 2.0 (Atlanta, Ga.: February 2010). Disease surveillance in livestock and poultry is a component of biosurveillance.

[4]Pub. L. No. 107–171, tit. X, subtit. E, §§ 10401-10418, 116 Stat. 494 (2002) (codified as amended at 7 U.S.C. §§ 8301-8317).

USDA on disease surveillance for influenza, a zoonosis that infects humans and some livestock and poultry.

Threats from biological agents, including zoonotic pathogens, highlight the need for an effective agricultural defense system, including disease surveillance in livestock and poultry. Animal disease surveillance consists of collecting, analyzing, and interpreting animal health data to detect diseases early, enable rapid reporting and response during disease outbreaks, and control the spread of disease.[5] As we reported in 2011, however, federal efforts in this regard are still in development: no centralized coordination effort is in place to oversee the federal agencies' overall implementation of Homeland Security Presidential Directive 9.[6] We also reported that the agency within the Department of Homeland Security designated to integrate national surveillance efforts does not receive from its federal partner agencies the kind of expertise it has identified as most critical for supporting its early-detection mission—particularly, data generated at the earliest stages of an event or outbreak.[7]

In this context, you asked us to review the federal government's efforts to conduct surveillance activities for animal diseases in livestock and wildlife. This report examines (1) USDA's new approach to disease surveillance in livestock and poultry in light of a changing disease landscape and challenges, if any, the agency faces with this approach and (2) the extent to which this approach is guided by a strategy with measurable goals and supports broader national biosurveillance efforts.

To address both these objectives, we reviewed presidential directives regarding biosurveillance, biodefense, and homeland security,

---

[5]GAO, *Biosurveillance: Developing a Collaboration Strategy Is Essential to Fostering Interagency Data and Resource Sharing*, GAO-10-171 (Washington, D.C.: Dec. 18, 2009).

[6]GAO-11-652.

[7]GAO-10-171.

specifically, Homeland Security Presidential Directives 7, 9, 10, and 21.[8] We also reviewed USDA's authorizing legislation, relevant regulations, guidance, policy documents, and strategic and other plans for disease surveillance in livestock and poultry, including the Animal Health Protection Act and the federal traceability rule for livestock moving between states. We interviewed officials from USDA and from the Departments of Health and Human Services, and Homeland Security who collectively have responsibilities for disease surveillance in livestock and poultry, surveillance for influenza and other zoonotic diseases, research, coordination of biosurveillance activities, and management of information technology used to track data on livestock and poultry diseases. We also reviewed USDA's disease surveillance planning documents, leading practices in strategic planning that we identified in prior work, and key strategic planning documents regarding national biosurveillance from the Departments of Health and Human Services, and Homeland Security. To review the issue in depth, we focused on disease surveillance in swine. We selected swine because they represent a significant portion of the nation's livestock and poultry industry and are susceptible to many diseases of national concern, including some that can sicken humans. In addition, USDA has initiated a comprehensive species surveillance program for swine, its first for livestock and poultry.

To collect information on specific disease surveillance practices, we selected four states for review: Colorado, Iowa, North Carolina, and Texas. We selected these states to ensure that our review (1) represented geographic variation in pork-producing regions; (2) included states with large swine populations, as well as states with comparatively smaller populations; and (3) represented a number of potential data sources for disease surveillance in livestock and poultry, such as livestock markets and veterinary diagnostic laboratories. Moreover, because feral swine present a potential source of infection to commercial food animal herds, we chose only states where feral swine

---

[8]Homeland Security Presidential Directive 7 establishes a national policy for federal agencies known as sector-specific agencies, which are responsible for particular industry sectors, such as transportation, energy, and communications, to identify and prioritize U.S. critical infrastructure and key resources and to protect them from terrorist attack; Homeland Security Presidential Directive 10 identifies actions to bolster the nation's biodefense capabilities; and Homeland Security Presidential Directive 21 establishes a national strategy for public health and medical preparedness that is aimed at transforming the nation's approach to protecting the health of the American people against all disasters.

are present.[9] Together, these four states represent 46 percent of the nation's commercial swine population. Because we did not select a generalizable sample of states, the results from these four states cannot be generalized to all states, but they can provide examples of disease surveillance practices in the four states. Within our four selected states, we obtained and reviewed state guidance on disease surveillance in livestock and poultry; forms the states use to obtain livestock and poultry health information for disease surveillance purposes; and strategic plans, where available. We also interviewed federal and state animal, public health, and veterinary laboratory authorities and pork producers or their representatives within our selected states; we also visited a hobby farm, a feral swine holding facility, and two livestock markets in most of these states. In addition, we interviewed representatives of the American Association of Veterinary Laboratory Diagnosticians, the American Association of Swine Veterinarians, the National Pork Board, and the National Pork Producers Council. We reviewed funding from fiscal year 2007 through fiscal year 2013 for USDA programs supporting disease surveillance in livestock and poultry, including funding to modernize information technology systems. We also reviewed annual reports for fiscal years 2010 through 2011 summarizing program data collected through USDA's Influenza in Swine Surveillance Program. These data include the number of biological submissions tested and the biological data analyzed. To assess the reliability of the financial data we analyzed, we reviewed USDA's agency financial reports for fiscal years 2009 to 2012 and relevant evaluations of USDA financial information by the USDA Office of Inspector General. We also interviewed budget officials to further confirm the data's accuracy. We identified no material problems with the accuracy of financial data reported by USDA. To assess the reliability of the influenza program data, we interviewed USDA officials familiar with how the data were collected, entered into the database, and checked for accuracy. We determined that the financial and program data were sufficiently reliable for our purposes.

We conducted this performance audit from November 2011 to May 2013 in accordance with generally accepted government auditing standards.

---

[9]The term *feral* refers both to domesticated animals that have escaped from domestication and become wild and to naturally wild animals descended from the same species as domesticated animals. While the Department of the Interior plays a critical role carrying out disease surveillance of wild animals, we did not include Interior's activities because they were beyond the scope of our review.

Those standards require that we plan and perform the audit to obtain sufficient, appropriate evidence to provide a reasonable basis for our findings and conclusions based on our audit objectives. We believe that the evidence obtained provides a reasonable basis for our findings and conclusions based on our audit objectives.

Background

According to international animal health authorities, disease surveillance in livestock and poultry has as its main purpose the early detection of diseases and disease outbreaks. It also plays an important role during outbreaks, such as monitoring how fast a disease is spreading through animal populations and in what direction. Disease surveillance is also critical in determining how effective efforts have been in controlling and eradicating disease from a particular area or animal population and in recognizing when that disease no longer poses an immediate threat to animal or human health. Further, surveillance supports international trade, allowing officials to certify that animals are healthy and safe to move across borders. Disease surveillance in livestock and poultry is particularly important because billions of cattle, swine, poultry, and other animals used for food are annually moved from place to place over long distances throughout the food supply chain—from wherever producers are located and then to feedlots and local, regional, and even overseas markets and slaughterhouses. Thus, to prevent the spread of contagious diseases and protect the welfare of healthy herds, animal health authorities often restrict the movement of animals. Such restrictions can lead, paradoxically, to the destruction of large numbers of uninfected animals and substantial economic losses.

Federal, state, tribal, and industry entities share responsibility for carrying out disease surveillance in livestock and poultry (see app. I).[10] Under the national animal health reporting system, APHIS typically works with states to monitor, control, and eradicate certain animal diseases. According to APHIS documents and state veterinary officials, such activities include, for example, issuing guidance on how to identify and report particular diseases of national concern, developing vaccination programs, and providing additional staff to work alongside state investigators tracking outbreaks of infectious diseases. To manage these reportable diseases,

---

[10]Throughout this report, we use the term *industry* to denote commercial producers of livestock and poultry.

APHIS has worked closely with the states and industry over the past decades to eradicate them by, for example, providing states funding and guidance. According to APHIS documents, the agency has made significant gains in eradicating reportable diseases such as tuberculosis and brucellosis, which have historically plagued American livestock. State animal health officials work closely with industry and with state-operated veterinary diagnostic laboratories to monitor and protect the health of livestock and poultry within state boundaries, including regulating the entry of livestock and poultry into their states. Veterinarians accredited under APHIS's National Veterinary Accreditation Program are directed to report to APHIS the suspected presence of selected domestic and foreign animal diseases that can cause significant economic, trade, or public health consequences (see app. II for a list of such diseases in swine).[11] Some states also require veterinarians to directly report to state animal health authorities the incidence of diseases that are not reportable nationally.

Industry is an important source of health data on livestock and poultry, privately maintaining that information and reporting it to state and federal officials when a reportable disease is suspected. Veterinarians working for livestock and poultry producers collect tissue and blood samples from animals and send them to a veterinary laboratory for diagnosis; these veterinarians are the first line of defense in disease surveillance, whether for detecting diseases or monitoring a disease during an outbreak. The laboratory returns test results confidentially to the veterinarian or person submitting the sample, unless the test results indicate the presence of a federal or state reportable disease, in which case those test results are reported to appropriate federal or state authorities. When a veterinarian suspects the presence of a foreign animal disease in a herd, the veterinarian contacts state and federal animal health authorities to take a sample and send it to APHIS's National Veterinary Services Laboratories to confirm the diagnosis (see fig. 1). If state and federal animal health officials approve, a National Animal Health Laboratory Network laboratory may conduct initial screening for certain foreign animal diseases. But a

---

[11]Under the National Veterinary Accreditation Program, APHIS approves veterinarians to perform certain official functions on its behalf. Veterinarians may perform duties only in the state within which they were accredited and maintain accreditation only as long as they comply with standards established in federal regulations, including reporting the suspected presence of certain animal diseases to APHIS. 9 C.F.R. pt. 161.

sample is also sent to APHIS's National Veterinary Services Laboratories to confirm the diagnosis.

Figure 1: How USDA Collects Information for Disease Surveillance from Livestock and Poultry Producers

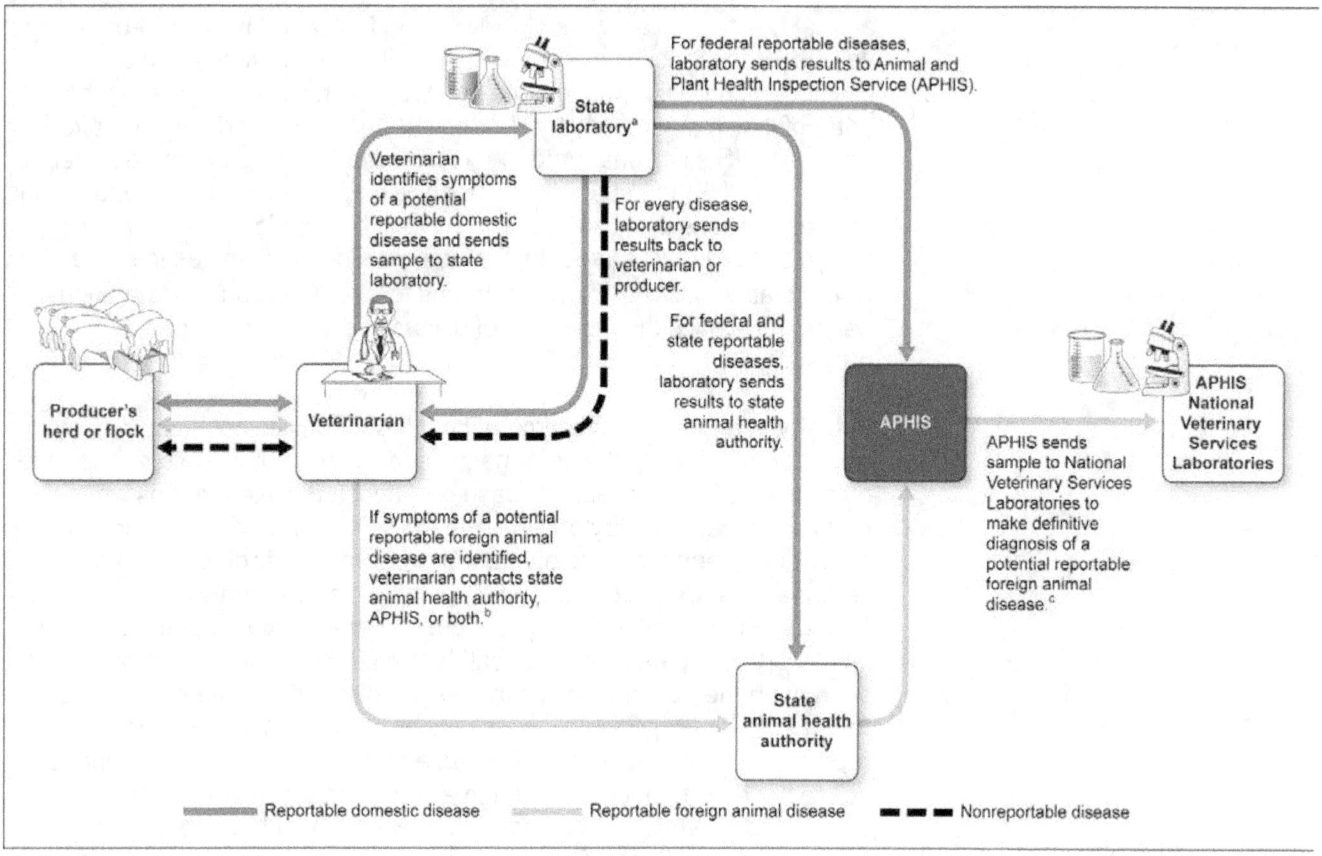

Source: GAO.

Note: Besides federally reportable diseases, states may monitor other diseases of interest that are reportable at the state level.

[a]Some state laboratories may be members of USDA's National Animal Health Laboratory Network and, as such, conduct routine diagnostic tests for domestic diseases and targeted surveillance tests for foreign animal diseases.

[b]The state animal health authority and APHIS assign a foreign animal disease diagnostician to collect and send a sample to the National Veterinary Services Laboratories.

[c]According to APHIS officials, a second sample may be sent to a National Animal Health Laboratory Network laboratory for preliminary diagnosis at the same time as a sample is sent to the National Veterinary Services Laboratories, which must confirm all diagnoses of these diseases.

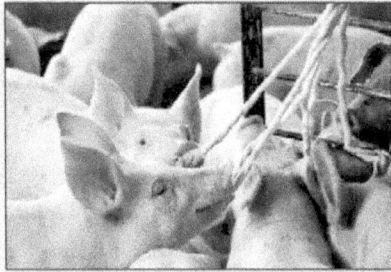
Contagious diseases with the potential to harm the economy and human health may spread among livestock and poultry, and in some cases be transmitted to humans, through various methods. For example, classical swine fever[12] may be transmitted from an infected swine to another directly through nose-to-nose and sexual contact or indirectly through a person or object, such as a farmhand's clothing. Swine may also contract the disease through exposure to or consumption of contaminated pork products, which typically occurs when swine are fed uncooked garbage or meat products from a source outside the United States. The classical swine fever virus is known to survive in pork meat for up to 180 days. Although this disease affects only swine, other diseases in swine have the capacity to affect humans. For example, swine can become infected not only with swine influenza viruses but with human and avian viruses as well. According to recent influenza research, evidence exists that influenza viruses can be transmitted through the air between swine and humans and that either host can be contagious before showing symptoms of illness. When a swine is infected with more than one influenza virus at the same time, the viruses can exchange genetic material, thereby creating a new influenza virus, which may vary in its virulence and transmissibility between and within species (see app. III).

---

[12]Classical swine fever is a highly contagious viral disease of swine not currently known to exist in the United States, which can cause major economic damage as a result of excessive animal illness, death, and trade restrictions.

USDA's APHIS Is Broadening Its Approach to Disease Surveillance in Livestock and Poultry and Faces Challenges in Doing So

To better adapt to the changing landscape of human and animal diseases (including the rapid global movement of humans, animals, and food products), APHIS has begun to shift its disease-specific surveillance approach to (1) monitor the overall health of livestock and poultry and (2) improve its ability to analyze health information about livestock and poultry. APHIS faces several challenges in carrying out this new approach, including obtaining new data from current and additional sources and determining how best to deploy declining resources, given increasing fiscal constraints.

APHIS's New Approach Monitors Overall Health of Livestock and Poultry and Seeks to Improve Collection and Analysis of Information

As funding for disease eradication programs changes, and the global landscape of animal and human diseases produces new threats, APHIS has since fiscal year 2012 begun broadening its previous disease-by-disease approach to one in which the agency monitors the overall health of certain livestock and poultry species. APHIS's intention is to examine the nation's livestock herds and poultry flocks in detail, using diverse sources of data, to better detect, monitor, and control diseases that may be new or reemerging, including domestic diseases of economic importance. Before its new approach, APHIS directed its programs for disease surveillance in livestock and poultry toward preventing the introduction of certain foreign animal diseases and to monitoring, detecting, and eradicating other reportable diseases already present in domestic herds. Information about nonreportable diseases, including diseases that were new or reemerging, was not always captured by the agency's disease surveillance efforts.

According to APHIS documentation, beginning in fiscal year 2010, the agency proposed its first effort to broaden disease surveillance in livestock and poultry: monitoring the health of the nation's hog, or swine, herds. This program—called Comprehensive and Integrated Swine Surveillance—identifies new sources and types of data on diseases in swine, among other things. Since fiscal year 2012, the agency has been receiving funding on a species, or commodity, basis, rather than on a disease-specific basis; thus, the agency's swine health activities, including surveillance, were provided dedicated funding for the first time that year at $23 million. To begin addressing multiple and evolving information needs about swine health under the program, the agency plans to draw new data from sites where swine typically converge in large numbers or where information on swine health can be easily collected. In planning documents, APHIS officials said that they plan to collect data from farms where swine are raised, markets where they are sold, slaughter facilities, and veterinary diagnostic laboratories, among other sites (see fig. 2). They also plan to collect data from feral swine, which may harbor diseases transmissible to domestic herds. Many of these sites are already monitored to some extent, but APHIS officials said they intend to expand how the sites are used in the future under the program. For example, APHIS has been monitoring for the presence of pseudorabies at slaughter facilities, but it has proposed monitoring these facilities for a range of other diseases as well, including classical swine fever.[13] According to agency officials, APHIS is also considering potential new information sources, such as data that states collect on diseases of regional concern, some of which fall outside the category of reportable diseases. APHIS has begun to take some of its planned actions under this program, but many of the planned actions require further coordination and concurrence from industry and states before they can be implemented.

Figure 2: Examples of Sources of Data on Swine Health

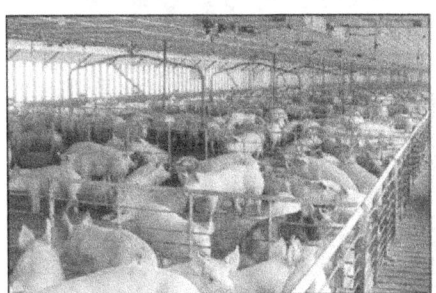

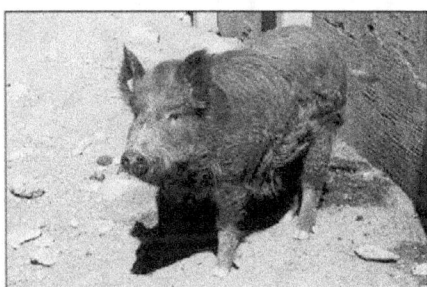

Sources: USDA and GAO.

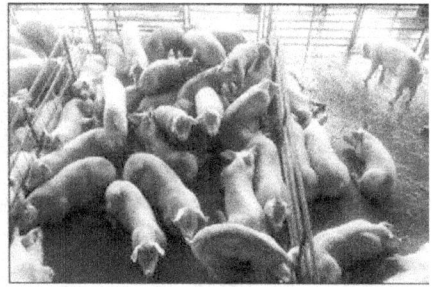

Commercial swine farm   Feral swine   Livestock market

In addition to making better use of existing data sources and identifying new ones, APHIS and the Department of Homeland Security launched a 9-month pilot program designed to use volunteer veterinarians to assist in detecting diseases early, including new and emerging diseases. Scheduled to conclude in May 2013, according to Homeland Security officials, this pilot program involves a number of participating private veterinarians, working in a small area of West Texas and New Mexico, who are using electronic tablets to record and submit to APHIS data on syndromes they observe in livestock herds, that is, data on the collective

---

[13]Pseudorabies is a viral disease of swine that may cause respiratory illness and death.

signs and symptoms of sickness that animals exhibit. According to a statement of work for this program, such information has not been systematically collected and reported before, and this pilot offers the opportunity to gauge the usefulness of such information.

Under this new approach, APHIS also plans to improve its ability to analyze information—collected from numerous sources for different purposes and in different formats—on the overall health of livestock and poultry, by standardizing how the information is reported and improving how the data are linked electronically. Because data standards vary greatly among APHIS's numerous information systems, and within individual systems, APHIS has limited ability to analyze and aggregate information to generate a complete national picture of livestock and poultry health. To address these limitations, APHIS in 2009 developed a multiyear information technology plan to restructure and modernize how the agency collects and manages information for detecting and monitoring diseases in livestock and poultry, including new and emerging disease threats. The technology plan's ultimate goal is to develop a centralized information repository containing health information about livestock and poultry from the most relevant internal and external databases and employing standardized data entry protocols.

The initial phase of this effort to improve efficiency and data analysis is already under way. APHIS in January 2013 replaced its outdated Generic Disease Database, which contained information on outbreaks of domestic diseases, with a new database management system, called Surveillance Collaboration Services, which establishes standardized data fields and codes. APHIS also plans to electronically link this new database system with, among others, its existing Emergency Management Response System, which contains information derived from investigations of suspected foreign animal diseases, and Laboratory Messaging Services, which receives and records diagnostic test results for selected diseases of national concern. Estimated at $5.4 million, the first phase of APHIS's technology modernization effort—the deployment of the Surveillance Collaboration Services system—is scheduled to be completed 1 year ahead of its original 2014 target date, APHIS officials said.

APHIS Faces Challenges Implementing Its New Approach

APHIS faces key challenges in carrying out this new approach to disease surveillance in livestock and poultry, in particular, gathering data from current and additional sources, such as from industry and from state animal health authorities, and determining how best to deploy declining resources.

Data

Obtaining new data on livestock and poultry health from current and additional sources is likely to be a challenge for various reasons, including (1) industry concerns over the confidentiality of animal health data and (2) the sufficiency of collected data.

Data Confidentiality

APHIS's ability to gather new data will likely be hindered by industry concerns that some health information on livestock and poultry should be kept confidential and not shared. For example, industry representatives and state animal health authorities we spoke with said they would not be willing to share information about the health of their herds beyond what is required by federal regulation because the information, including information on the incidence of influenza in swine, might be made public and affect sales. These officials cited as an example a 2009 H1N1 influenza outbreak in humans, which was genetically linked to an influenza virus found in swine and led to millions of dollars in lost sales to the pork industry because people mistakenly believed they could become ill from eating pork. Moreover, state animal health officials from one state reported that their state laws prohibit them from releasing information they collect on the health of their state's livestock and poultry unless the information is required to be reported by federal law to control an immediate threat to overall animal or public health.

Moreover, APHIS may have difficulty obtaining complete data identifying individual livestock and poultry and their locations. Generally, the states, not the federal government, maintain animal identification and location data, in part because of industry data confidentiality concerns, according to APHIS documents. APHIS officials told us that most states will share this information during animal disease outbreaks, but some do not routinely share the information for surveillance purposes. This reluctance to routinely share could affect the agency's ability to generate a national picture of diseased and at-risk animals and their locations—information essential to effectively monitor and control livestock and poultry diseases, including new and emerging diseases. In July 2007, we reported that, for a number of reasons, APHIS faced serious challenges implementing a comprehensive national animal identification system.[14] In January 2013,

---

[14]GAO, *National Animal Identification System: USDA Needs to Resolve Several Key Implementation Issues to Achieve Rapid and Effective Disease Traceback*, GAO-07-592 (Washington, D.C.: July 6, 2007).

APHIS published a rule establishing national standards for identifying animals and documenting their movement that, with some exceptions, made it mandatory for livestock and poultry under federal regulation that are moved across state lines to have official identification and documentation. The new rule addresses some limitations of the old system, giving states some discretion in administering the program, including managing information required and maintained on animals entering their borders.

The flexibility given to states with regard to how they maintain animal identification information under the new rule also poses challenges for APHIS to obtain information effectively and in a standardized manner. For example, states may use APHIS's approved types of animal identification, including animal identification numbers, and approved official documentation, such as the interstate certificate of veterinary inspection, but they can also use alternative systems. An APHIS document on animal disease traceability says that although states can use a number of animal identification systems, they must follow certain standards, but states need not abide by APHIS's suggested standards for documentation. In addition, states may track data in APHIS's animal identification and movement information systems or may maintain their own databases instead, and these databases may not be compatible with APHIS's systems. According to APHIS officials, standards are being developed to ensure future compatibility.

Data Sufficiency

APHIS will likely face the challenge of gathering sufficient data to monitor diseases, because agency officials and pork producers differ in their views on how much collected information is enough to successfully identify potential disease threats. For example, APHIS officials reported that commercial producers voluntarily and anonymously shared nearly 9,400 swine samples with APHIS's National Swine Influenza Virus Surveillance Program in 2012, a 72 percent increase over the 5,460 samples submitted in 2011. But agency officials and pork producers disagree somewhat about whether collected data are sufficient to allow the program to successfully identify potential disease threats. About 66 million swine are raised on 68,300 U.S. farms. Agency animal and human health researchers have questioned whether enough swine samples and information are being submitted to APHIS's influenza surveillance program. Influenza researchers also explained to us that because the data are submitted anonymously and cannot be linked with a particular farm or herd, they cannot be sure that the samples commercial producers provide to APHIS are representative of the viruses currently circulating domestically. Several pork producers, in contrast, told us they believe that the data APHIS has collected have been sufficient.

APHIS also faces the challenge of obtaining sufficient data to monitor serious diseases that could spread to domestic herds and people from the nation's sizable and widespread feral swine population. Federal and state animal health officials and pork producers told us that feral swine pose a significant risk because they carry diseases that have been eradicated in domestic herds, such as brucellosis and pseudorabies, which, if reintroduced, could hinder hog movement and trade. According to APHIS documents, feral swine are also susceptible to contracting and transmitting foreign animal diseases because they are highly mobile, at times crossing the border with Mexico and eating out of landfills, where they might encounter contaminated garbage. The introduction of a foreign animal disease like classical swine fever could close export markets. Feral swine are also carriers of zoonotic diseases, such as brucellosis and influenza, which can infect humans and other species. Feral swine are most likely to affect small backyard farms with little security, but they may also attempt to infiltrate larger, more secure operations.

Unlike domestic herds, feral swine are not easily accessible to veterinarians and wildlife biologists responsible for managing populations and monitoring diseases, and, according to federal and state officials, even when feral swine are located, they can be very difficult to capture. In addition, the population is growing rapidly. According to APHIS data, feral swine were present in 36 states as of 2010, their population distribution and range having increased from 28 states in 2004 and 17 states in 1982 (see fig. 3). Officials from APHIS's Wildlife Services told us that they have been sampling approximately 3,000 feral swine per year and testing for various diseases, including influenza, pseudorabies, brucellosis, and classical swine fever. Nevertheless, given an estimated nationwide population of 5 million feral swine, officials said that they would need to test significantly more animals per year to accurately portray the extent of diseases in this population.

Figure 3: Expansion of Nationwide Feral Swine Population, 1982, 2004, and 2012

Instructions: Move mouse over individual years in the legend below to reveal the related swine distribution. For a printable version of this figure, see appendix V.

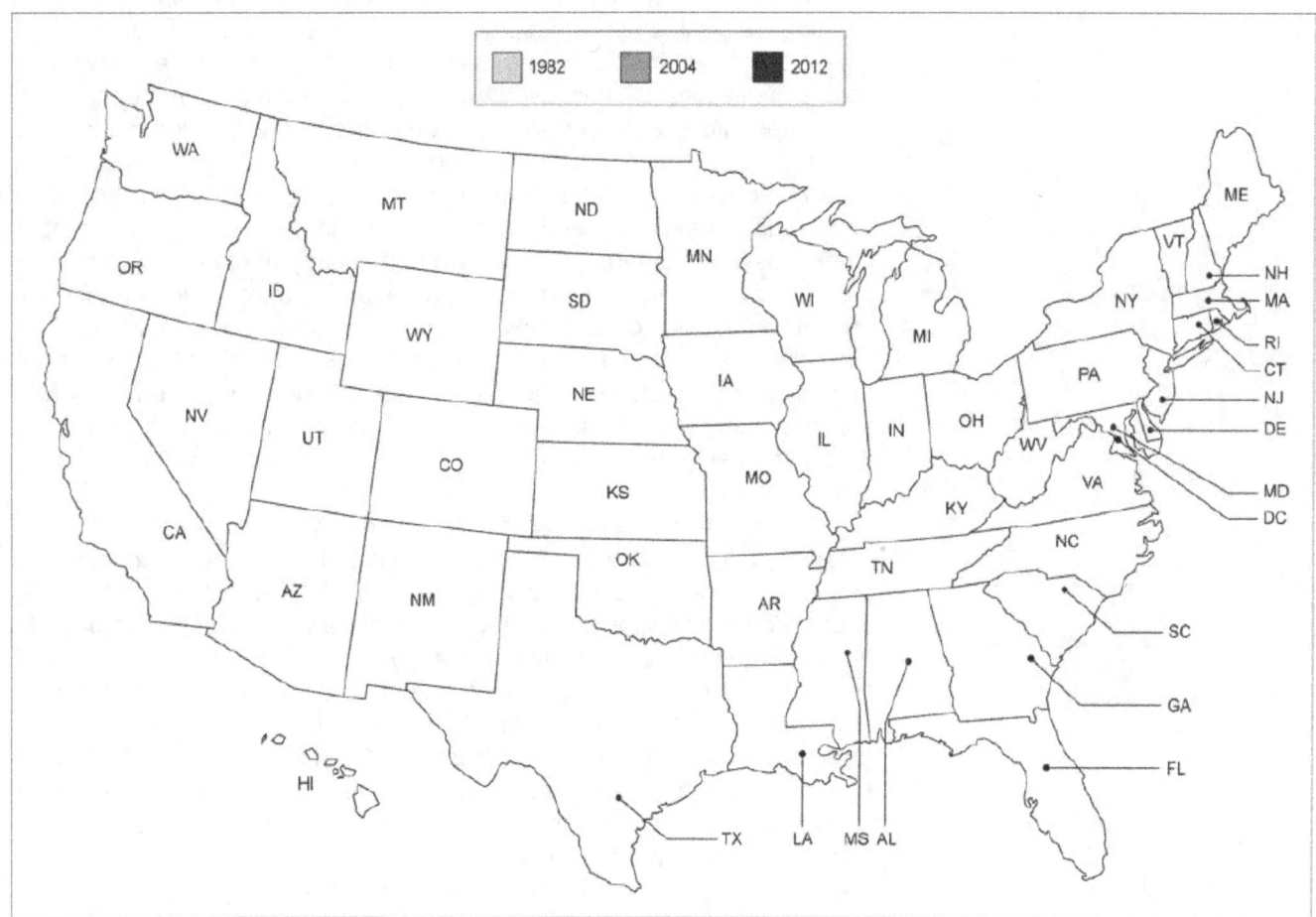

Sources: GAO analysis of USDA and state wildlife agency data; copyright © Corel Corp., all rights reserved (map).

Note: According to APHIS officials, although most of the feral swine population within specific areas in the earlier years remained there in later years, control efforts had removed some feral swine from a few small areas by 2012.

Resources

Declining resources—funding constraints and a shortage of veterinarians—also pose a challenge to broadening disease surveillance and improving analysis of livestock and poultry health data, according to APHIS officials.

Funding Constraints

Federal and state animal health officials told us that decreased funding to USDA is a challenge to APHIS's disease surveillance efforts in livestock and poultry. According to agency documentation, the budget for APHIS recently decreased by about 14 percent for fiscal years 2008 through 2013. As a result, APHIS has seen funding for key components of its disease surveillance efforts decline as well, according to agency officials. For example, funding for federal-state cooperative agreements for monitoring animal health has decreased by 44 percent, from $46 million in 2009 to $25 million in 2012.[15] We previously reported that state officials in agriculture and wildlife departments said that they depend largely or completely on federal funds to support biosurveillance efforts and that their capabilities to carry out disease surveillance and other biosurveillance activities would be limited without funding from federal grants and cooperative agreements.[16] Funding for APHIS's National Wildlife Disease Surveillance and Emergency Response System, responsible for disease surveillance in feral swine, has been reduced by 71 percent, or $16 million, from fiscal year 2006 to fiscal year 2012. Additionally, funding for other disease surveillance programs has declined or remains uncertain. For example, the Department of Health and Human Services provided a one-time $25.75 million in funding to APHIS in 2009 to extend the agency's prevention and surveillance capabilities for influenza virus in swine.[17] Because of a recent increase in the number of

[15]The decrease was due in part to the removal in 2011 of targeted funding from APHIS's appropriation and the reduction in 2012 of funding for certain diseases, which affected funding for some cooperative agreements.

[16]GAO, *Biosurveillance: Nonfederal Capabilities Should Be Considered in Creating a National Biosurveillance Strategy*, GAO-12-55 (Washington, D.C.: Oct. 31, 2011).

[17]In 2009, the Department of Health and Human Services transferred $27.75 million in supplemental funding to USDA to fund the agency's capabilities to prepare for and respond to pandemic influenza after the 2009 novel H1N1 influenza A outbreak. Of that funding, APHIS received $25.75 million for prevention and surveillance activities, and the Agricultural Research Service received $2 million to develop improved prevention and detection tools.

GAO-13-424 Disease Surveillance in Livestock and Poultry

submitted samples from swine, however, APHIS officials project that funding will run out by fiscal year 2015 or earlier. As a result, APHIS officials said, the agency might not be able to continue to offer stakeholders viral diagnostic testing or genetic sequencing services using this funding. USDA officials told us they are uncertain whether future funding will exist for these activities.

In addition, state officials participating in USDA's National Animal Health Laboratory Network have reported that insufficient and declining funding is reducing their ability to effectively and rapidly identify, report, and respond to an outbreak of a serious disease, such as foot-and-mouth disease. For example, officials from member laboratories have reported difficulties maintaining essential diagnostic personnel and expertise. The network receives funding from APHIS for operational support, including testing, equipment maintenance, training assays, and travel. APHIS and USDA's National Institute of Food and Agriculture also provide support for infrastructure, including personnel and maintaining and developing information technology. According to APHIS officials, funding from APHIS to pay for testing for certain diseases has decreased even though overall funding has increased somewhat since 2007. In addition, funding for laboratory infrastructure provided by the National Institute for Food and Agriculture has declined by 40 percent. Laboratory officials told us that this drop forced some laboratories to cut their staffing levels, reducing the number of highly trained personnel who can perform the biological tests needed to rapidly identify, report, and respond to diseases. Member laboratory officials also told us that working with an outdated National Animal Health Laboratory Network information system limited the efficiency with which data generated from laboratory testing can be transmitted to APHIS.

Shortages of Veterinarians

According to federal and state officials, a decrease in the number of APHIS field veterinarians has also reduced the agency's ability to carry out critical disease surveillance activities effectively. At the time of our review, officials in each of the four states we visited reported a reduced number of field veterinarians as a primary challenge to effective collection of health data from livestock and poultry. Some officials explained that, in particular, too few veterinarians affected veterinarians' ability to stay in frequent contact with farms, such as small farms having little biosecurity and a high risk of their animals' contracting serious diseases. For example, officials in one state reported a vacant position for the state's primary APHIS field veterinarian. Another state official reported that even as livestock and poultry imports have increased—with the number of swine entering the state increasing on average by about 1 million per year from 2002 to 2011—the number of field veterinarians responsible for coordinating disease surveillance across 99 counties decreased from 11 in 2001 to 7 in 2012. Such declines are symptomatic of a more general decline in the number of veterinarians, particularly livestock and poultry veterinarians. In 2009, for example, we reported that four of the five key agencies that employ veterinarians—USDA's APHIS, Food Safety and Inspection Service, and Agricultural Research Service and the Army—identified existing or potential shortages in the federal veterinary workforce, which agencies have begun to address, including by participating in the Office of Personnel Management's veterinary medical officer advisory council to address the shortage.[18]

No Overall Strategy with Goals and Measures Guides APHIS's New Approach to Animal Disease Surveillance

APHIS has a vision for its new approach but has not integrated that vision into an overall strategy with associated goals and performance measures aligned with the nation's larger biosurveillance efforts. None of APHIS's planning documents clearly define (1) the goals the agency wants to achieve in the long term with its new disease surveillance approach, (2) how the agency intends to measure results, or (3) how APHIS's disease surveillance efforts support national biosurveillance efforts.

No Overall Disease Surveillance Strategy with Goals and Measures Ties APHIS's Various Plans Together

APHIS has a number of planning documents that describe a new strategic vision and mission for the primary division responsible for the agency's new disease surveillance approach. Nevertheless, the agency has not integrated that vision into an overall strategy with associated goals and measures supporting the nation's larger biosurveillance efforts. The Government Performance and Results Act, as amended, requires federal agencies to develop performance plans that include measurable goals.[19] We have previously reported that these requirements can also serve as leading practices for planning at lower levels within agencies,

---

[18]GAO, *Veterinarian Workforce: Actions Are Needed to Ensure Sufficient Capacity for Protecting Public and Animal Health*, GAO-09-178 (Washington, D.C.: Feb. 4, 2009).

[19]Government Performance and Results Act, Pub. L. No. 103-62 (1993), 107 Stat. 285, amended by GPRA Modernization Act of 2010, Pub. L. No. 111-352, 142 Stat. 3866.

such as individual divisions, programs, or initiatives.[20] Developing goals and performance measures helps an organization balance competing priorities, particularly if resources are constrained, and helps an agency assess progress toward intended results. Long-term strategic goals unify an agency's many efforts in a coordinated framework for achieving results. Goals should correspond to the purposes set forth in the agency's mission statement, they should cover the major functions and operations of an agency, and they should be measurable. Developing goals and performance measures helps an organization address important dimensions of program performance, balances competing priorities— especially if resources are declining or constrained—and shows progress or contributions to intended results. Performance measures, which typically have numerical targets, are important management tools that help an agency identify the activities that work well and those that do not. Without such performance measures, agencies cannot determine whether the activities and programs they are carrying out are accomplishing the goals they intend to achieve.

A number of APHIS planning documents (see app. IV for a list of selected planning documents) describe a new strategic vision and mission for APHIS's Veterinary Services organization—the primary division responsible for implementing the new disease surveillance approach. Veterinary Services' planning documents acknowledge that in preventing and detecting diseases in livestock and poultry and protecting animal health, the agency plays an important role in safeguarding public and environmental health as well. The goals APHIS has identified in these planning documents focus primarily on processes or activities but do not specifically address outcomes the agency seeks to accomplish or have associated performance measures. For example, the principal planning document explaining the agency's future vision and mission includes the following goals: transforming the culture of the organization, investing in technical infrastructure, and supporting readiness and response.[21] These goals describe what actions the agency intends to undertake but not what

---

[20]GAO, *Homeland Security: Agriculture Inspection Program Has Made Some Improvements, but Management Challenges Persist,* GAO-12-885 (Washington, D.C.: Sept. 27, 2012).

[21]USDA Animal and Plant Health Inspection Service, *Veterinary Services: A New Perspective* (Washington, D.C.: 2011).

GAO-13-424 Disease Surveillance in Livestock and Poultry

outcomes these actions are intended to achieve or how the agency will measure intended results.

Agency officials said that in the past, when APHIS focused its activities primarily on selected reportable diseases, measuring success was relatively straightforward: a primary performance measure of program success was the extent to which specific diseases had been eradicated and prevented from entering the United States or—in the case of eradicated diseases—prevented from reemerging. For example, APHIS's animal disease programs have largely eradicated brucellosis in cattle and brucellosis and pseudorabies in domestic commercial U.S. swine; in addition, reentry of foot-and-mouth disease has been prevented: the nation has been free of foot-and-mouth disease since 1929. Officials we interviewed expressed concern, however, that traditional outcome measures like these may no longer be valid when applied to newly emerging diseases. For example, new influenza viruses, which may affect human health, are already circulating in domestic livestock and mutate so effectively that eradication is not considered possible.

The principal planning document for Veterinary Services establishes a goal to enhance the health of the nation's animals by "anticipating and responding to new or emerging threats" but also states that the agency must still develop an effective mechanism for evaluating such threats and determining an appropriate response.[22] Other, more-detailed Veterinary Services planning documents primarily communicate the key steps and obstacles to implementing a new approach to disease surveillance.[23] They define issues—such as the need to develop better relationships with stakeholders—and identify potential ways of addressing these issues, but they do not tie the issues to an outcome-based goal or offer performance measures for gauging progress. In sum, none of these planning documents provide APHIS with a clear road map or overall strategy, with associated performance measures, for managing its new approach to animal disease surveillance.

---

[22]USDA Animal and Plant Health Inspection Service, *Veterinary Services Strategic Plan FY 2006 to FY 2011* (Washington, D.C.: undated).

[23]USDA Animal and Plant Health Inspection Service, *Veterinary Services 2015 Project: Surveillance for Action Strategic Direction* (Washington, D.C.: 2011) and Centers for Epidemiology and Animal Health, National Surveillance Unit, "Implementation of Comprehensive and Integrated Swine Surveillance," (Fort Collins, Co., Jan. 22, 2010).

Without performance measures, APHIS cannot construct the necessary relevant indicators of performance that ultimately reveal if the activities or initiatives the agency is pursuing—such as the collection of influenza data from swine—are the right ones and being carried out effectively. Given that influenza researchers are unsure to what extent the data collected from swine are sufficient or representative of the viruses circulating domestically, measurable goals could better enable the agency to demonstrate progress or success with the data they have already collected or intend to collect. But without specific measures of the outcomes APHIS intends to accomplish in following the behavior of novel diseases, the agency cannot, among other things, assess the utility of the data it is collecting or determine if it needs data sources other than those it has already identified. Neither can APHIS weigh its activities against one another to give higher priority to funding activities with the greatest potential to benefit animal and human health. APHIS, state animal health authorities, and publicly funded veterinary diagnostic laboratories all face increasing constraints on resources, which has, according to agency officials, impeded efforts to modernize information technology systems; monitor herd health; and efficiently and effectively test samples for animal diseases.

APHIS officials said that they recognize a need for adequate goals and reliable performance measures focused on outcomes. Indeed, officials said they have plans to develop goals and performance measures for their new approach but that under increasing fiscal pressure—APHIS's budget decreased about 14 percent from fiscal year 2008 through fiscal year 2013—they have focused first on streamlining operations, improving efficiencies, and carrying out already-funded pilot disease surveillance programs. For example, APHIS has proposed restructuring how business units within Veterinary Services are organized across the services' field offices and headquarters and to modernize information technology systems. According to veterinary officials, their proposed actions achieve cost efficiencies over time, as well as support a broader approach to monitoring the health of livestock and poultry. In addition, the deputy administrator of Veterinary Services said, several new disease surveillance initiatives—including the pilot program to collect animal health data remotely in the field on mobile electronic devices and another to collect and test samples submitted voluntarily by producers and samples taken from swine at slaughter—can help determine both the quality of, and ease of access to, new sources of disease surveillance data. Once these initiatives and pilots have been implemented and evaluated, he said, he believes APHIS will be better situated to develop the goals and performance measures needed to determine the success of their new and broader approach to animal disease surveillance. APHIS officials did not provide a time frame for developing goals and measures.

These efforts would certainly help inform APHIS's development of meaningful goals and performance measures, but resource constraints—and the risk that the introduction of a new or reemerging disease may substantially harm animal and human health—suggest it would be prudent for APHIS to move forward quickly to develop performance measures focused on outcomes to guide their disease surveillance efforts. As the results of APHIS's surveillance initiatives become clearer, the agency can adjust its approach accordingly.

APHIS's Plans Do Not Define Their Relationship with the Nation's Biosurveillance Efforts

None of APHIS's various plans indicate how they individually or collectively support national homeland security efforts called for in Homeland Security Presidential Directive 9, or additional biosurveillance efforts that together make up a national policy to defend the nation's food and agricultural systems against terrorist attacks, major disasters, and other emergencies. The goals cited in these APHIS planning documents do not mention homeland security or tie an APHIS goal to a national biosurveillance effort. On the one hand, APHIS, in collaboration with the Department of Homeland Security's National Center for Foreign Animal and Zoonotic Disease Defense, has developed an Emergency Response Support System (or "information dashboard"). This system aims to bring together multiple potential sources of disease information on livestock and poultry—from federal and state governments, producers, and current research—into a single coordinated and integrated system to complement the Department of Homeland Security's broader effort to support a national biosurveillance system. The Emergency Response Support System was developed by the Foreign Animal and Zoonotic Disease Center at Texas A&M University and funded with help from the department.[24] According to Disease Center officials, this information dashboard is intended to provide APHIS and its stakeholders the ability to quickly call up and display relevant sources of animal disease information and to nationally map producers' farms, disease outbreaks, and animal movement, among other patterns, onto a computer monitor. On the other

---

[24]According to Department of Homeland Security budget documents, the department has invested $2.2 million in developing a national web-based software platform to support what it calls a biosurveillance common operating picture. APHIS's Emergency Response Support System is to be one component of that larger system.

hand, however, none of the planning documents we reviewed indicates how this information dashboard is to align with or support broader national-level biosurveillance efforts.

Similarly, the planning documents make no mention of coordinating with other homeland security efforts to enhance disease surveillance in livestock and poultry. For example, the Department of Homeland Security has provided funding to develop tools for disease surveillance, such as an assay that tests swine saliva for foreign animal diseases, which can test samples from more than one animal at a time and may be faster and easier than collecting tissue or other biological samples. Officials involved in developing such diagnostic tools, however, told us that responsibilities shared between APHIS and the department have sometimes complicated development and use of such tools. As we have previously reported, federal agencies can use their strategic and annual performance plans as tools to drive collaboration with other agencies and partners and establish complementary goals and strategies for achieving results.[25] Thus, an absence of shared measurable goals between APHIS and the Department of Homeland Security may be compromising both agencies' understanding of how their monitoring of animal health—coupled with disease surveillance, control, and eradication efforts—complement broader national biosurveillance goals. APHIS officials agreed that it is important for the agency's planning documents to show how the agency's efforts support national homeland security efforts to enhance the detection of biological threats.

Conclusions

APHIS has long carried out important work to protect the nation's livestock and poultry against economically devastating infectious diseases and against the potential deadly effects of such diseases on people. Foot-and-mouth disease has not infected cattle or swine in the United States since 1929, and pseudorabies and brucellosis have been virtually eradicated in commercial swine and cattle. The near elimination of tuberculosis is considered one of the greatest animal and public health achievements in the United States. Moreover, given the changing disease landscape, APHIS has begun to craft a more comprehensive approach to monitoring animal health—one no longer restricted to eradicating only

---

[25]GAO, *Agencies Need Better Collaboration to Reduce the Risk of Animal Related Diseases*, GAO-11-9 (Washington, D.C.: Nov. 8, 2010).

certain diseases. We commend the agency for its efforts (1) to develop a vision for its new approach and planning documents for undertaking it and (2) to collect better data from new and different sources and better synthesize and analyze information to identify potentially harmful new pathogens earlier. Nevertheless, APHIS has not to date developed goals or performance measures for its new approach; agency officials said they have plans to do so, but they did not provide a time frame. Even with its efforts to date, however, without integrating the vision in its planning documents into an overall strategy with associated goals and measures that are aligned with broader national homeland security efforts to detect biological threats, APHIS may not be ideally positioned to support national efforts to address the next threat to animal and human health.

Recommendation for Executive Action

As APHIS develops goals and measures for its new approach to disease surveillance in livestock and poultry, we recommend that the Secretary of Agriculture direct the APHIS Administrator to integrate the agency's vision into an overall strategy, with associated goals and measures, that guides how APHIS's new approach will support national homeland security efforts to enhance the detection of biological threats.

Agency Comments and Our Evaluation

We provided a draft of this report for review and comment to the Departments of Agriculture, Health and Human Services, and Homeland Security. USDA and the Department of Homeland Security provided written comments, which are reproduced in appendixes VI and VII, respectively; these agencies also provided technical comments, which we incorporated as appropriate. The Department of Health and Human Services had no comments.

In its written comments, USDA concurred with our recommendation that APHIS integrate the agency's vision into an overall strategy that guides how APHIS's new approach will support national homeland security efforts. USDA stated that APHIS will include better performance metrics in its planning efforts and develop more explicit linkages between its swine surveillance activities and other national homeland security efforts.

In its letter, the Department of Homeland Security thanked us for the opportunity to review the draft report and noted that the department supports developments at APHIS to advance disease surveillance in animal and plant populations. The Department of Homeland Security also stated that it remains committed to working with its many partners, including those in the federal government, to better mitigate and defend against dynamic threats and maximize the ability to respond to and recover from attacks and disasters of all kinds.

We are sending copies of this report to the Secretaries of Agriculture, Health and Human Services, and Homeland Security; appropriate congressional committees; and other interested parties. In addition, the report is available at no charge on the GAO website at http://www.gao.gov.

If you or your staff members have any questions regarding this report, please contact me at (202) 512-3841 or garciadiazd@gao.gov. Contact points for our Offices of Congressional Relations and Public Affairs may be found on the last page of this report. Key contributors to this report are listed in appendix VIII.

Daniel Garcia-Diaz
Director
Natural Resources and Environment

Appendix I: Key Stakeholders in Disease Surveillance in Livestock and Poultry

Table 1 lists the primary federal, state, and private-sector organizations or groups that have a key role or stake in the surveillance of diseases in livestock and poultry. The list includes animal health organizations, human health organizations concerned with zoonotic diseases that might be transmitted between livestock and poultry and humans, and those organizations interested in monitoring diseases in livestock and poultry as part of broader national biosurveillance efforts.

Table 1: Key Stakeholders in Disease Surveillance in Livestock and Poultry

Lead organization	Agency	Subagency	Role	Surveillance-related responsibilities
		Federal		
Animal health				
U.S. Department of Agriculture (USDA)	Agricultural Research Service		Research to improve agricultural production	Veterinarians and scientists in the Agricultural Research Service do research to support diagnostic testing, vaccines, disease management systems, and farm biosecurity measures, among other tools, to help national efforts to detect, control, and eradicate animal diseases of national priority.
	Animal and Plant Health Inspection Service (APHIS)		Lead agency for animal health surveillance	APHIS is responsible for implementing and conducting national measures to detect, control, or eradicate any livestock and poultry disease (such as drawing blood and diagnostic testing), including in animals at slaughterhouses, stockyards, or other points of concentration. The agency develops new and improves existing national strategies and technologies for dealing with intentional and unintentional introduction of animal diseases.
		Veterinary Services	National veterinary authority	Veterinary Services is the office within APHIS that manages the nation's livestock disease surveillance, control, and eradication efforts. The office oversees the agency's surveillance planning, management, diagnosis, and analytical efforts to identify and respond to animal disease incidents.

Lead organization	Agency	Subagency	Role	Surveillance-related responsibilities
		Center for Veterinary Biologics	Regulation of biological products for diagnosis, prevention, or treatment of animal diseases	The Center for Veterinary Biologics monitors and inspects biological products, including vaccines and diagnostic tests, to ensure that they are free of disease-producing agents, especially foreign animal diseases. It also tests the effectiveness of, and issues licenses and permits for the commercial use of, these products.
		National Animal Health Laboratory Network	National coordination of state-level veterinary diagnostic laboratories	The National Animal Health Laboratory Network connects and supports state-level member veterinary diagnostic laboratories with funding, infrastructure, training, common testing methods, and software platforms, among other things, to provide a national capacity to quickly and efficiently respond to and report animal disease outbreaks.
		National Veterinary Services Laboratories	National veterinary diagnostic support and reference laboratories	The National Veterinary Services Laboratories diagnose domestic and foreign animal diseases of national concern. They are the only laboratories in the nation with the capacity to confirm the presence of a foreign animal disease. The laboratories support USDA's disease control and eradication programs and provide training and assistance to veterinary diagnostics laboratories nationwide. As the nation's reference laboratories, they form the center of expertise and guidance on diagnostic techniques.
	Wildlife Services		Wildlife damage management and research authority	Wildlife Services, through its operational program and the National Wildlife Research Center, employs veterinarians, biologists, and epidemiologists to research and mitigate damage caused by wildlife to public health and safety, agriculture, and natural resources, including diseases in wildlife.

Lead organization	Agency	Subagency	Role	Surveillance-related responsibilities
	Food Safety and Inspection Service		Regulation of commercial animal products	Food Safety and Inspection Services inspectors conduct surveillance of livestock and meat and poultry products in slaughter facilities around the country, looking for symptoms or abnormalities that could indicate presence of a disease.
	National Institute of Food and Agriculture		Support of agricultural research, education, and extension programs	The National Institute of Food and Agriculture supports and funds agricultural research, education, and extension programs. One of the programs it supports is the National Animal Health Laboratory Network, through programmatic leadership and funding for personnel, training, and infrastructure.
Human health				
Department of Health and Human Services (HHS)	Centers for Disease Control and Prevention (CDC)		Lead agency for human health surveillance	CDC develops strategies for conducting surveillance of diseases in humans, including coordinating with USDA and other agencies to monitor zoonotic diseases.
		National Center for Immunization and Respiratory Diseases, Influenza Division	National human influenza surveillance center	The Influenza Division of the National Center for Immunization and Respiratory Diseases conducts surveillance of influenza in humans, including human infections of influenza of animal origin. Researchers use surveillance information to monitor influenza trends and improve rapid reporting and identification of novel influenzas of animal origin to which humans might not have immunity. Researchers also use surveillance to guide the development of diagnostic tests and vaccines.

Lead organization	Agency	Subagency	Role	Surveillance-related responsibilities
	National Institutes of Health		National medical research agency	The National Institutes of Health is made up of 27 research institutes and centers, including the National Library of Medicine, which houses over 200 databases, including GenBank, a genetic sequence database that provides the scientific community access to the most updated and comprehensive DNA sequence data related to diseases of concern.
Biosurveillance coordination				
Department of Homeland Security	Office of Health Affairs		Lead agency for national biosurveillance coordination	The Office of Health Affairs provides medical, public health, and scientific expertise in support of the Department of Homeland Security's mission to prepare for, respond to, and recover from all threats. It serves as the principal advisor to the Secretary of Homeland Security and the Administrator of the Federal Emergency Management Agency on medical and public health issues.
		National Biosurveillance Integration Center	Coordination of information to support national biosurveillance capability	The National Biosurveillance Integration Center collects and analyzes reports from federal partners, including USDA and CDC, of incidents and outbreaks of diseases of national concern. The center then develops and provides synthesized reports and updates to the White House, federal partners, and state and local stakeholders on potential biosecurity threats, through analyzing aggregated information for animal disease, human disease, and environmental quality surveillance.
		Food, Agriculture, and Veterinary Defense Division	Coordination of national activities to protect agriculture and animal health	The division provides expertise and consultation to the Department of Homeland Security to help secure the nation's food, agriculture, and veterinary public health systems against potential threats.

Lead organization	Agency	Subagency	Role	Surveillance-related responsibilities
	Science and Technology Directorate		Research and development of products and technology solutions to support homeland security activities	The Science and Technology Directorate provides science and technology research support to the Department of Homeland Security; strengthens the ability of communities to respond to disasters; and identifies and develops appropriate technologies to counter chemical, biological, and other threats to national security.
	Zoonotic and Animal Disease Defense Center of Excellence		Consortium of universities advancing animal health research	Established in 2010, the Zoonotic and Animal Disease Defense Center of Excellence is composed of the Foreign Animal and Zoonotic Disease Center at Texas A&M University and the Center of Excellence for Emerging and Zoonotic Disease at Kansas State University. These institutions share responsbilities to conduct research on foreign animal, emerging, and zoonotic diseases; develop countermeasures to these diseases; and develop models and information analysis tools. The Department of Homeland Security provides funding and oversight.
State				
State or university-based member veterinary diagnostic laboratories	National Animal Health Laboratory Network member laboratories		Animal disease diagnostic services	Network member laboratories provide expertise to identify animal disease incidents by performing routine diagnostic testing and monitoring diseases of concern. The laboratories conduct diagnostic testing in response to requests by individual veterinarians and producers and also to support federal targeted surveillance programs for selected domestic and foreign animal diseases to prevent and help control the spread of these diseases.

Lead organization	Agency	Subagency	Role	Surveillance-related responsibilities
State departments of agriculture	State veterinarians		Principal state animal health official	State veterinarians provide services to support and regulate the health of livestock and poultry within their state boundaries. State veterinarians coordinate surveillance, detection, and reporting of diseases within their states. They maintain a list of reportable diseases that threaten the health of livestock, require accredited veterinarians to report disease occurrences, and then report these occurrences to USDA. These officials work with federal veterinarians in the prevention, detection, and eradication of selected domestic and foreign diseases associated with national animal disease programs.
State departments of health	State public health veterinarian		Animal health liaison to state public health official	State public health veterinarians monitor, investigate, and control zoonotic diseases in humans to protect public health.
Private sector				
Livestock and poultry industry	Livestock and poultry owners and producers		Producers monitor the health of their flocks and herds, treat for illnesses, and vaccinate as necessary	Livestock and poultry owners and producers regularly observe the health of their herds and flocks to diminish disease introduction, including monitoring for specific clinical signs. They work with private veterinarians to collect biological samples to test for diseases routinely or as needed when animals become ill. The data collected are normally proprietary and used to enhance and protect production, unless they pertain to a disease that is regulated and must be reported to USDA.

Source: GAO analysis of USDA and state documents and information.

Appendix II: Status of Reportable Swine Diseases in the United States, 2011

Table 2 shows the status in the United States of swine diseases that are to be reported to the Department of Agriculture's (USDA) Animal and Plant Health Inspection Service (APHIS) when they are confirmed to be present in swine.[1]

Table 2: Status of Reportable Swine Diseases in the United States, 2011

Disease	Description	Affects humans?	Status
African swine fever	A viral disease endemic in Africa. The virus is highly contagious, spreading by direct and indirect contact, and persists for long periods both in pork products and in the environment. Forms of this virus vary in virulence from highly pathogenic forms that cause near 100 percent mortality to low-virulence forms that can be difficult to diagnose. No vaccine or treatment is available.	No	Free[a]
Anthrax	A bacterial disease found most commonly in wild and domestic herbivores, such as cattle, sheep, and goats. It can also infect humans exposed to infected animals, animal products, or spores of the anthrax bacterium. Rapid onset of respiratory and other symptoms are typical in cattle and sheep, which often die shortly after symptoms appear. Infected humans may experience sores on the skin's surface, intestinal discomfort, and influenza-like symptoms, which may cause death. Vaccines are available.	Yes	Present
Aujeszky's disease (pseudorabies)	A viral disease found in swine that kills piglets and produces a lifelong infection in older pigs. It does not affect humans. Swine may transmit the disease to other species, such as cattle, sheep, cats, and dogs. In other animals, the disease causes intense itching and death. Vaccines are available.	No	Present
Brucellosis	A bacterial disease found most commonly in swine, cattle, and bison. The disease is transmitted by direct contact with infected animals or with bodily fluids of infected animals. The primary symptoms of the disease are abortion in pregnant animals and lower fertility rates. Infected humans suffer severe intermittent fever. Vaccines are available.	Yes	Present
Classical swine fever	A highly contagious viral disease of both commercial and feral swine, also known as hog cholera. Although not now found in the United States, the disease is found in Mexico. Pigs are infected through nose-to-nose and sexual contact or indirectly through a person or object, such as a farmhand's clothing. The disease results in fever, loss of appetite, diarrhea, and hemorrhages of the skin and may cause death. In breeding herds, the disease produces abortions. Vaccines are available but do not allow animal health officials to distinguish between infected and vaccinated animals.	No	Free

[1]These diseases are also reportable to the World Organisation for Animal Health, formerly known as the Office International des Epizooties (OIE). The organization adopted its present name in May 2003 and has kept its historical abbreviation OIE.

Disease	Description	Affects humans?	Status
Echinococosis, or hydatidosis	An emerging parasitic zoonosis originating in eastern European and Asian countries caused by a tapeworm found in dogs, sheep, cattle, goats, and pigs. It produces harmful, slowly enlarging cysts in the liver, lungs, and other organs; can be undetected for many years; and may be fatal. No vaccines are available.	Yes	Presence suspected but not confirmed
Foot-and-mouth disease	A highly contagious disease that affects cloven-hoofed animals, including swine, cattle, sheep, and deer. It does not affect humans. Although infected animals usually survive, they are afflicted with fever and blisterlike lesions on the tongue, lips, and feet that cause severe debilitation. Nations where this disease is present face strict livestock export restrictions. Vaccines are available, although no one universal vaccine is effective against all forms, and it is difficult for animal health officials to distinguish between infected and vaccinated animals.	No	Free
Japanese encephalitis	A serious viral disease found primarily in Asia and transmitted by mosquitoes to both animals and humans. Illness ranges from mild symptoms of fever and lethargy to severe brain infection. The disease can cause reproductive problems in pigs. Pigs and birds can have large numbers of viruses in their blood and serve as a major reservoir of the virus. One in four persons infected with Japanese encephalitis dies; others suffer permanent brain damage. A vaccine is available.	Yes	Free
Leptospirosis	A zoonotic disease caused by infection with a spirochete bacterium; about 200 variations of spirochete bacteria have been identified. Clinical signs vary but include abortions, stillbirth, weak piglets, and infertility. Accurate diagnosis is difficult. Vaccines are available but may not provide solid immunity. In humans, the disease can be lethal. No vaccines are available.	Yes	Present
New World screwworm	A parasitic infection of screwworms, which are blowfly larvae (maggots) that feed on living flesh, usually on superficial wounds or mucous membranes. The parasites infest all mammals, rarely birds. Before its eradication from North and Central America, the disease caused devastating losses among livestock and wild animals. No vaccine is available.	Yes	Free
Nipah virus encephalitis	A highly contagious, emerging disease that originates in bats and causes encephalitis and death in humans and neurological symptoms in livestock, including swine, making it a serious public health concern. Transmission to humans is generally through contact with contaminated tissues of pigs and other livestock that have been infected through bat urine or saliva. No vaccine is available.	Yes	Free
Old World screwworm	Similar to New World screwworm, but the parasites are a different type of blowfly.	Yes	Free
Porcine cysticercosis	A parasitic infection of tapeworms, which invade a host's intestinal tract, muscles, brain, and other tissue, causing neurological, visual, and other physiological problems. The parasites are spread when humans or pigs consume undercooked meat or come in contact with flies. Vaccines are available.	Yes	Absent during 2011 reporting period

Disease	Description	Affects humans?	Status
Porcine reproductive and respiratory syndrome	A viral disease first identified in the 1980s and widespread globally at present, the syndrome is characterized by respiratory distress in swine and lowered birth rates, abortions, stil births, and weak infants. Not all affected swine display symptoms. Vaccines are available.	No	Present
Rabies	A viral disease of the central nervous system of mammals, including feral swine, which involves an extremely high mortality rate. Vaccines can protect pets, as well as people exposed to these animals, but the maintenance of rabies viruses in wildlife complicates control.	Yes	Present
Rinderpest	A viral disease of cattle sometimes called cattle plague. Rinderpest can also infect buffalo, feral swine, goats, and sheep. Most susceptible are cattle, which suffer from diarrhea, dehydration, and fever and often die.	No	Free
Swine vesicular disease	A viral disease clinically indistinguishable from foot-and-mouth disease. This disease produces vesicles, or ulcers, on the coronary bands (where the skin and hide join with the hoof); heels; and occasionally on the lips, tongue, snout, and teats. Severe cases occur where pigs are housed on abrasive floors in damp conditions. No vaccine is available.	No	Free
Transmissible gastroenteritis	A highly infectious viral disease in piglets caused by a corona virus. Provokes vomiting and diarrhea. The disease destroys villi—small fingerlike structures—in the small intestine. Mortality can be 100 percent in newborn piglets. Vaccines are available, but results have been variable.	No	Present
Trichinellosis	A parasitic infection of adult worms in the small intestine of host species, including pigs, humans, and other flesh-eating mammals. The worms plant their larvae in the hosts' muscle tissue. The disease is transmitted to humans in raw or undercooked meat from infected livestock or game. This disease can cause influenza-like symptoms and weakness and lead to death in humans. In animals, the infection is often unapparent. No vaccine exists.	Yes	Presence suspected but not confirmed
Tularemia	A bacterial disease spread by infected animals, through the air and by ingestion, ticks, and deer flies. Also called rabbit fever, tularemia occurs naturally worldwide and is considered a potential biological weapon. The disease can display from mild to severe influenza-like symptoms in humans and animals. No vaccine is available.	Yes	Present

Source: GAO analysis of USDA documents and information.

Note: The year 2011 is the last year for which data were available from APHIS.

[a]The term "free" refers to the absence of a disease, meaning that the disease has been eradicated or never existed in a particular location.

Appendix III: Creation of a Novel Human Influenza Virus in 2011

When influenza viruses reproduce, they can exchange gene segments in a process known as reassortment—a genetic shuffling—that can create new influenza viruses containing gene segments that may have originated in different host animals. In 2011, the Centers for Disease Control and Prevention (CDC) confirmed 12 cases of a novel influenza virus called an H3N2 variant virus, and in 2012, 309 cases of this virus were reported.[1] The genetic makeup of this virus showed that it was derived from (1) a virus that had been circulating in swine and (2) the human H1N1 virus that caused the 2009 influenza pandemic. Thanks to still earlier genetic shuffling, the gene segments in this novel 2011 influenza virus came from humans, birds, and swine, as illustrated in figure 4.

---

[1]According to CDC, influenza viruses that normally circulate in pigs are called "variant" viruses when they are found in humans. A USDA official said that APHIS had detected the H3N2 group of viruses in 2010 and confirmed the viruses' ability to infect and circulate among swine before human infections were reported in 2012.

GAO-13-424 Disease Surveillance in Livestock and Poultry

Interactive Graphic   Figure 4: Creation of a Novel Human Influenza Virus in 2011

Instructions: Move mouse from left to right over blue arrow in lower left in order to see how the segments from the existing viruses combine to create the 2011 human H3N2 variant virus. For a printable version of this figure, see appendix V.

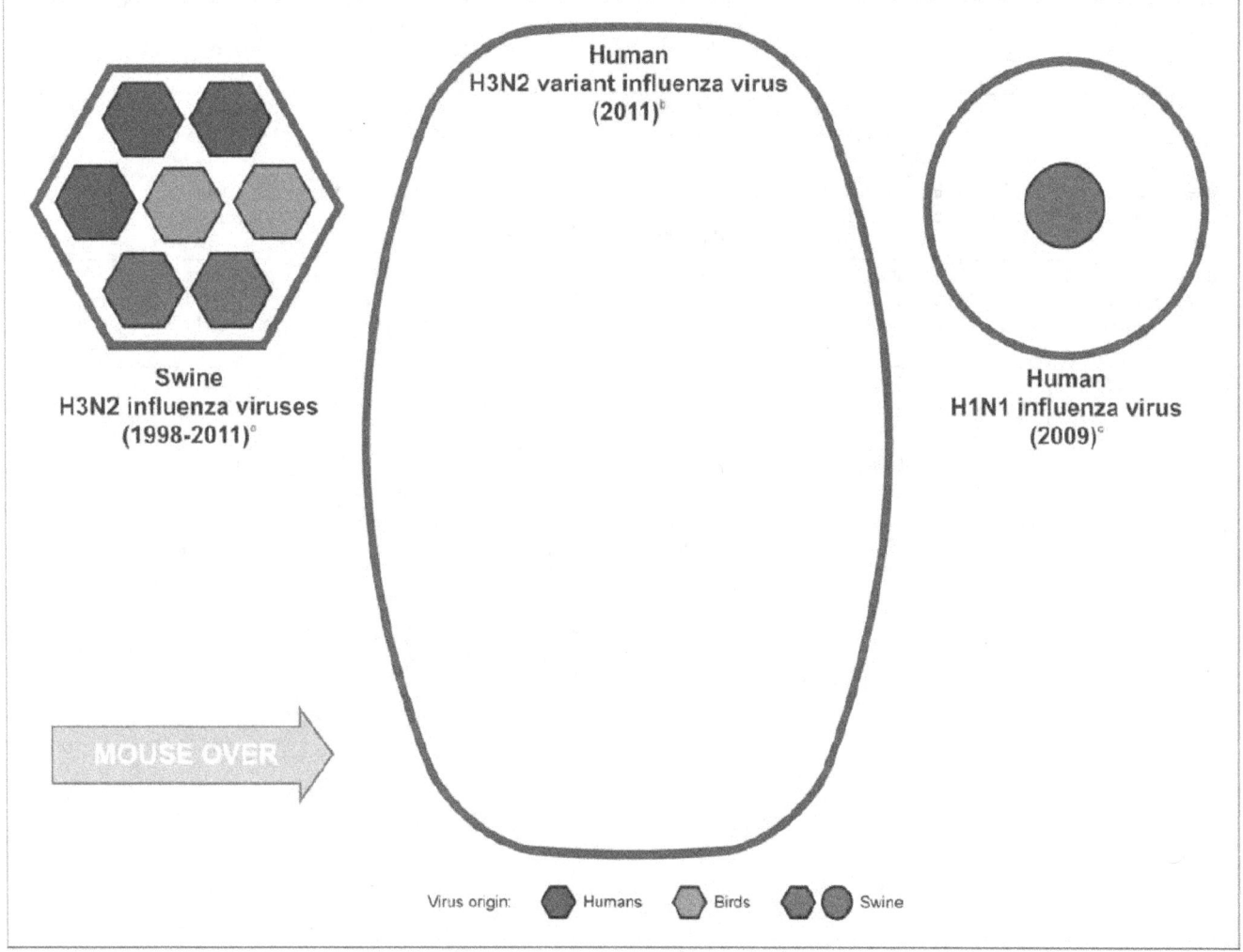

Sources: GAO and Centers for Disease Control and Prevention.

[a]From 1998 to 2011, H3N2 influenza viruses were identified in U.S. swine that possessed gene segments derived from human, avian, and swine viruses.

[b]In 2011, CDC confirmed 12 human cases of a novel H3N2 influenza variant virus containing one gene segment from the human H1N1 virus responsible for the 2009 pandemic (circle) and other gene segments from the H3N2 virus that had been circulating in swine from 1998 through 2011 (hexagons). These gene segments in turn had their origins in humans (blue) and birds (green), as well as swine (raspberry).

[c]In spring 2009, an H1N1 influenza virus of swine origin caused a worldwide pandemic in humans. The virus was subsequently passed back to swine, infecting animals worldwide.

Appendix IV: List of Selected APHIS Plans Related to Disease Surveillance in Livestock and Poultry

Plan name	Key characteristics	Date
Veterinary Services Strategic Plan FY 2006 to FY 2011[a]	Recognizes potential bioterrorism threats, as well as naturally occurring threats to the health of animals, and establishes goals and objectives to monitor for and protect against these threats; does not include performance measures	Undated
Veterinary Services: A New Perspective	Establishes a new strategic vision and mission for APHIS's Veterinary Services, recognizing that in preventing and detecting animal diseases and protecting animal health, the agency also plays an important role in safeguarding the health of people and the environment	Undated
The Secure Pork Supply Plan	Proposal to establish controls and procedures that will allow swine to continue to move between production facilities and processing plants in the event of an outbreak of a foreign animal disease	2011
Veterinary Services 2015 Project: One Health Strategic Direction	Establishes general goals and indicators of success for improving the global health of people, animals, ecosystems, and society but nothing specific to the new surveillance approach in livestock and poultry	2011
Veterinary Services 2015 Project: Surveillance for Action Strategic Direction	Recommends steps to move APHIS away from a disease eradication surveillance approach to a more comprehensive animal health surveillance approach, such as collecting a wider range of data from a greater variety of sources to improve the ability to detect and control emerging diseases	2011
Implementation of Comprehensive and Integrated Swine Surveillance	Proposal to move away from surveillance activities focused on eradicating specific diseases of swine to a focus on activities that monitor overall swine health	2010
National Surveillance Plan for Swine Influenza Virus in Pigs	Establishes objectives, sampling methods, and procedures for collecting and analyzing genetic information on influenza viruses found in commercial swine	2010
The Information Technology Roadmap	Establishes a plan to modernize APHIS's animal disease information systems, ensure data security, electronically link key data systems, and create standards for data entry	2009

Source: GAO analysis of USDA information.

Note: This table lists planning documents that USDA's Veterinary Services and we identified as key to surveillance. USDA's planning documents also include several documents that provide guidance on foreign animal disease preparedness and response, such as plans to address highly pathogenic avian influenza, foot-and-mouth disease, classical swine fever, and emerging disease incidents.

[a]FY = fiscal year.

Appendix V: Printable Interactive Graphics

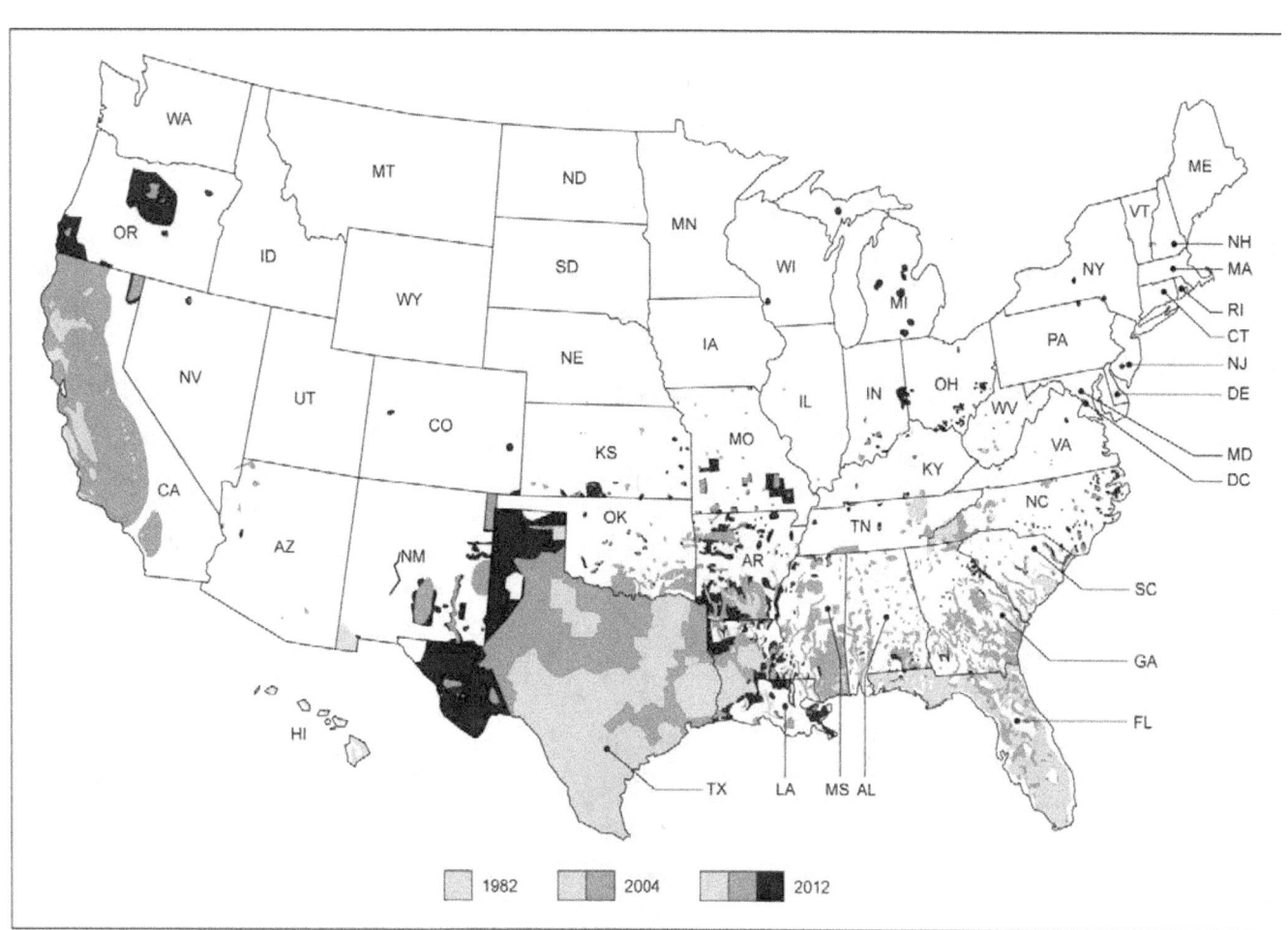

Sources. GAO analysis of USDA and state wildlife agency data; copyright © Corel Corp., all rights reserved (map).

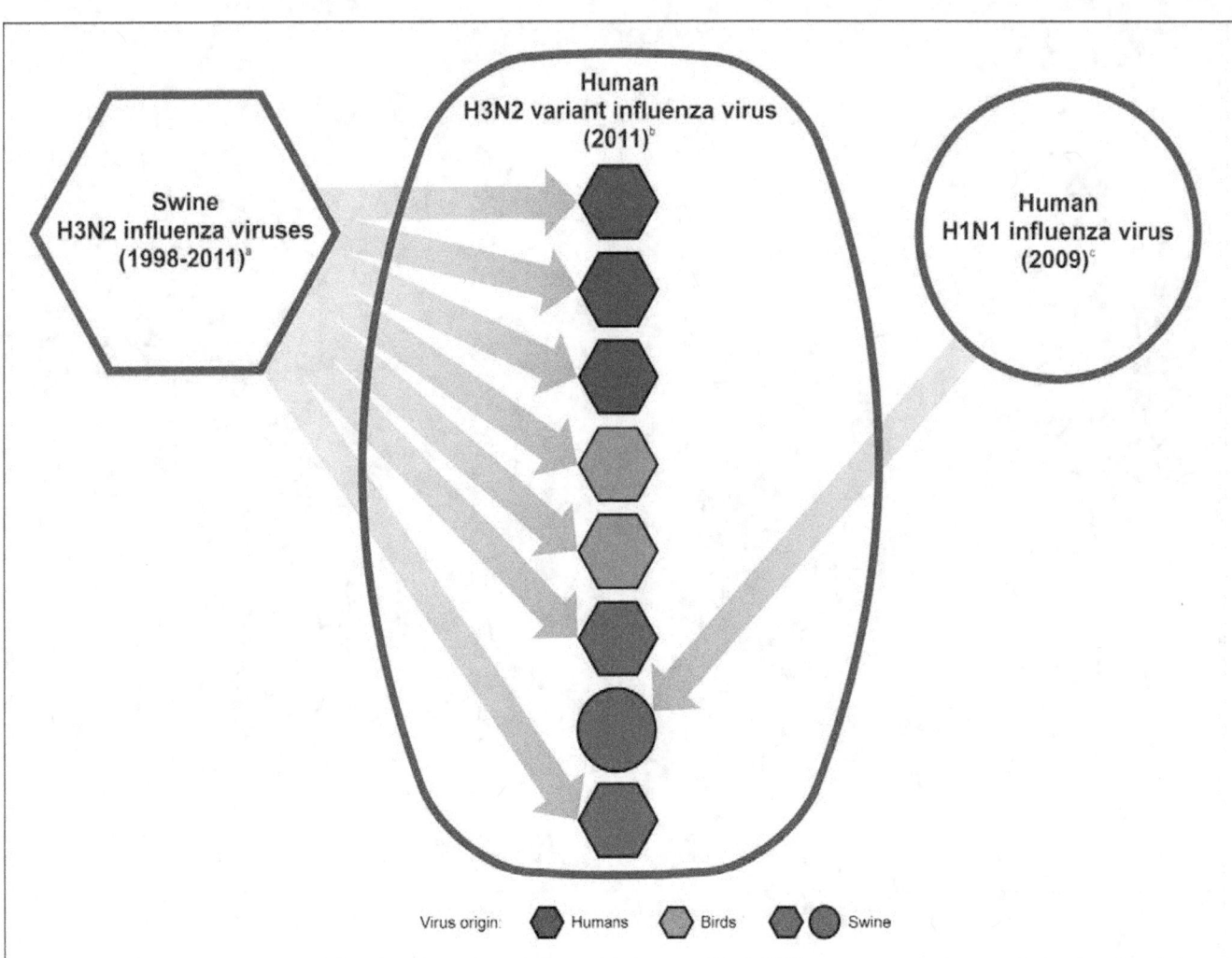

Sources: GAO and Centers for Disease Control and Prevention.

Appendix VI: Comments from the Department of Agriculture

United States Department of Agriculture

Office of the Secretary
Washington, D.C. 20250

APR 2 9 2013

Mr. Daniel Garcia-Diaz, Director
Natural Resources and Environment Issues
Government Accountability Office
441 G Street NW
Washington, DC 20548

The United States Department of Agriculture (USDA) appreciates the opportunity to review and comment on the GAO's Draft Report titled "Homeland Security: An Overall Strategy Is Needed to Strengthen Livestock and Poultry Disease Surveillance" (13-424). We have addressed the Recommendation for Executive Action.

GAO Recommendation

As APHIS develops goals and measures for its new approach to disease surveillance in livestock and poultry, we recommend that the Secretary of Agriculture direct the APHIS Administrator to integrate the agency's vision into an overall strategy, with associated goals and measures, that guides how APHIS's new approach will support national homeland security efforts to enhance the detection of biological threats.

USDA Response

USDA concurs with this recommendation. USDA's Animal and Plant Health Inspection Service (APHIS) is developing and implementing its new surveillance approach on a commodity-by-commodity basis. APHIS has produced numerous planning documents guiding its vision for a National Animal Health Surveillance System, and also has a strategy for Comprehensive and Integrated Swine Surveillance. APHIS will include better performance metrics in its planning efforts. For example, in the next twelve months, APHIS will develop performance measures for its Comprehensive and Integrated Swine Surveillance. Further, APHIS will also develop more explicit linkages between its swine surveillance activities and the National Strategy for Biosurveillance (signed by the President 7/31/2012), the Interagency Policy Committee called the Disaster Resilience Group's (DRG) implementation of the National Strategy for Biosurveillance, and the surveillance activities described in the Homeland Security Presidential

An Equal Opportunity Employer

Mr. Daniel Garcia-Diaz, Director
Page 2

Directive (HSPD-9). In the future, as APHIS develops new surveillance plans for the other
commodities, performance measures will be incorporated into those plans.

Sincerely,

Edward Avalos
Under Secretary
Marketing and Regulatory Programs

Appendix VII: Comments from the Department of Homeland Security

U.S. Department of Homeland Security
Washington, DC 20528

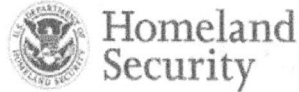

April 24, 2013

Daniel Garcia-Diaz
Director, Natural Resources and Environment Issues
U.S. Government Accountability Office
441 G Street, NW
Washington, DC 20548

Re: Draft Report GAO-13-424, "HOMELAND SECURITY: An Overall Strategy Is Needed to
Strengthen Livestock and Poultry Disease Surveillance"

Dear Mr. Garcia-Diaz,

Thank you for the opportunity to review and comment on this draft report. The U.S. Department of
Homeland Security (DHS) appreciates the U.S. Government Accountability Office's (GAO's) work
in planning and conducting its review and issuing this report.

DHS understands the importance of and supports the need to strengthen surveillance practices for
livestock and poultry disease. Within the Department, the National Biosurveillance Integration
Center's (NBIC's) primary mission is to enhance the capability of the Federal Government to rapidly
identify, characterize, localize, and track a biological event of national concern. NBIC strives to
achieve this by integrating and analyzing data relating to human health, animal, plant, food, and
environmental monitoring systems, both nationally and internationally. NBIC also disseminates
alerts and other information to Member Agencies and, in coordination with them, to other agencies of
state, local, and tribal governments, as appropriate, to enhance the ability of such agencies to respond
to a biological event of national concern.

NBIC supports developments at the U.S. Department of Agriculture (USDA) Animal and Plant
Health Inspection Service to advance disease surveillance in animal and plant populations. NBIC is
actively engaged with USDA to advance national directives and policies, including those related to
Homeland Security Presidential Directive 9. DHS remains committed to working with its many
partners – including those across the Federal Government, public and private sectors, and
internationally – to strengthen the Homeland Security enterprise to better mitigate and defend against
dynamic threats, minimize risks, and maximize the ability to respond to and recover from attacks and
disasters of all kinds.

We noted the report does not contain any recommendations specifically directed to DHS; however,
we thank you for the opportunity to review and comment on this draft report. Technical comments
were previously provided under separate cover. Please feel free to contact me if you have any
questions. We look forward to working with you in the future.

Sincerely,

Jim H. Crumpacker
Director
Departmental GAO-OIG Liaison Office

Appendix VIII: GAO Contact and Staff Acknowledgments

GAO Contact	Daniel Garcia-Diaz, (202) 512-3841 or garciadiazd@gao.gov.
Staff Acknowledgments	In addition to the contact named above, Mary Denigan-Macauley (Assistant Director), Kevin Bray, Ellen W. Chu, Kirsten Lauber, Dan Royer, Kiki Theodoropoulos, Ginny Vanderlinde, and Karen Villafana made key contributions to this report.

GAO's Mission	The Government Accountability Office, the audit, evaluation, and investigative arm of Congress, exists to support Congress in meeting its constitutional responsibilities and to help improve the performance and accountability of the federal government for the American people. GAO examines the use of public funds; evaluates federal programs and policies; and provides analyses, recommendations, and other assistance to help Congress make informed oversight, policy, and funding decisions. GAO's commitment to good government is reflected in its core values of accountability, integrity, and reliability.
Obtaining Copies of GAO Reports and Testimony	The fastest and easiest way to obtain copies of GAO documents at no cost is through GAO's website (http://www.gao.gov). Each weekday afternoon, GAO posts on its website newly released reports, testimony, and correspondence. To have GAO e-mail you a list of newly posted products, go to http://www.gao.gov and select "E-mail Updates."
Order by Phone	The price of each GAO publication reflects GAO's actual cost of production and distribution and depends on the number of pages in the publication and whether the publication is printed in color or black and white. Pricing and ordering information is posted on GAO's website, http://www.gao.gov/ordering.htm. Place orders by calling (202) 512-6000, toll free (866) 801-7077, or TDD (202) 512-2537. Orders may be paid for using American Express, Discover Card, MasterCard, Visa, check, or money order. Call for additional information.
Connect with GAO	Connect with GAO on Facebook, Flickr, Twitter, and YouTube. Subscribe to our RSS Feeds or E-mail Updates. Listen to our Podcasts. Visit GAO on the web at www.gao.gov.
To Report Fraud, Waste, and Abuse in Federal Programs	Contact: Website: http://www.gao.gov/fraudnet/fraudnet.htm E-mail: fraudnet@gao.gov Automated answering system: (800) 424-5454 or (202) 512-7470
Congressional Relations	Katherine Siggerud, Managing Director, siggerudk@gao.gov, (202) 512-4400, U.S. Government Accountability Office, 441 G Street NW, Room 7125, Washington, DC 20548
Public Affairs	Chuck Young, Managing Director, youngc1@gao.gov, (202) 512-4800 U.S. Government Accountability Office, 441 G Street NW, Room 7149 Washington, DC 20548

www.ingramcontent.com/pod-product-compliance
Lightning Source LLC
Chambersburg PA
CBHW080618290526
45790CB00007B/2829